EPIC EATS

EAT RIGHT, LIVE EPIC

2023

DOBBS MEDIA

Table of Contents

1. Understand Your Nutritional Needs

Understanding your nutritional needs is the cornerstone of a healthy eating journey. It's akin to having a map that guides you on a trek; the clearer your map, the smoother your journey. Two fundamental aspects of this map are calories and macronutrients. Delving deeper:

- **Calories:**

Calories are the energy units that our food provides and our body uses for its various functions. From the beating of your heart to the lifting of your fingers, everything costs energy.

  - **Determining Caloric Needs:** Your daily calorie requirement isn't a one-size-fits-all number. It's influenced by several factors:

    - **Age:** Generally, as we age, our metabolic rate slows down, leading to reduced caloric needs.

- **Gender:** Typically, men tend to have more muscle mass than women, leading to slightly higher caloric requirements.

- **Physical Activity:** A sedentary person will need fewer calories than someone who's more active.

- **Health Status and Special Conditions:** Conditions like pregnancy, illnesses, or recovery phases can influence caloric needs.

To get an estimate of your daily caloric needs, you can use online calculators, apps, or consult with a nutritionist. However, remember that these are just starting points. Listening to your body's hunger and fullness cues is crucial.

- **Macronutrients:**

Macronutrients are the major nutrients that form the bulk of our diet and provide us with energy. They are:

- **Carbohydrates:** The body's primary source of energy. They break down into glucose in our system and fuel our day-to-day activities. Sources include grains, fruits, and legumes.

  - **Types:** Simple carbs (sugars) provide quick energy but can cause energy crashes. Complex carbs (like whole grains) provide sustained energy.

  - **Recommendation:** About 45-65% of your total daily calories should ideally come from carbohydrates, primarily from whole sources.

- **Proteins:** The building blocks of the body, essential for repair, growth, and maintenance. They consist of amino acids, some of which are termed "essential" because our body can't produce them.

  - **Sources:** Meat, dairy, legumes, and some grains and vegetables.

  - **Recommendation:** Roughly 10-35% of your daily calories should come from proteins. Ensure a good mix of sources to get all essential amino acids.

- **Fats:** Vital for cellular functions, protecting organs, and aiding in nutrient absorption. Though dense in calories, they're essential for health.

  - **Types:** Unsaturated (good fats found in nuts, seeds, fish, and oils), saturated (found in animal products, can be consumed in moderation), and trans fats (artificial and harmful).

  - **Recommendation:** About 20-35% of your daily intake should be fats, predominantly from unsaturated sources.

In summary, understanding and balancing your caloric and macronutrient intake lays a strong foundation for a healthful dietary pattern. It's the first step in taking charge of your nutrition and crafting a diet that's both pleasurable and beneficial.

2. Eat a Variety of Foods

Variety is often referred to as the "spice of life," and when it comes to nutrition, this adage holds immense significance. A diversified diet doesn't just make your meals more enjoyable but also ensures that your body receives a mix of different nutrients essential for its optimal functioning. Let's delve deeper into the importance and benefits of a varied diet:

Why is Variety Essential?

- **Nutrient Spectrum:** Different foods come packed with varied nutrients. No single food contains all the essential vitamins, minerals, and antioxidants we need. Hence, rotating between food groups ensures we harness the benefits of each.

- **Digestive Health:** A diverse range of foods can contribute to a healthier gut. Fiber from various plant sources promotes healthy bowel movements and feeds the beneficial bacteria in our gut, fostering a robust microbiome.

- **Disease Prevention:** Regularly consuming a mix of foods can lower the risk of chronic diseases. For instance, different colored fruits and vegetables contain various types of antioxidants, each with unique health benefits.

- **Palate Pleasure:** A varied menu keeps your meals interesting, making it more likely for you to stick to healthy eating habits in the long run.

How to Incorporate Variety:

- **Vegetables:** Aim for a "rainbow" approach. Each color signifies a different set of nutrients. For instance:

  - *Green* (spinach, broccoli) offers vitamins like folate and vitamin K.

  - *Red* (tomatoes, bell peppers) often has lycopene, linked to heart health.

  - *Purple* (eggplant, beets) are rich in anthocyanins, known for their antioxidant properties.

- **Fruits:** Just like with vegetables, diversity is key. Citrus fruits like oranges and lemons are Vitamin C powerhouses, while berries bring in a host of antioxidants and apples provide dietary fiber.

- **Grains:** Move beyond just wheat and rice. Experiment with quinoa, barley, millets, and oats. Each grain has its own nutrient profile. For instance, quinoa is a complete protein, while oats are known for their heart-healthy properties.

- **Protein Sources:** Diversity in protein sources ensures you get a range of amino acids.

  - *Animal-Based:* Rotate between poultry, fish, eggs, and lean meats. Fish, especially fatty varieties like salmon, provide omega-3 fatty acids essential for brain health.

  - *Plant-Based:* Beans, lentils, tofu, chickpeas, and tempeh are excellent protein sources. They're also packed with other nutrients like fiber, iron, and magnesium.

Tips for Enhancing Variety:

1. **Explore New Recipes:** A new recipe can introduce you to foods you haven't tried before.

2. **Seasonal Eating:** Seasonal foods are not only fresher but also diversify your diet throughout the year.

3. **Ethnic Cuisine:** Trying dishes from various cultures can introduce you to a myriad of ingredients.

4. **Shop Differently:** Every once in a while, buy a fruit, vegetable, or grain you've never had before. It's a simple step towards diversification.

In conclusion, eating a variety of foods isn't just a dietary recommendation—it's a strategy for holistic health, ensuring that our body gets a symphony of nutrients working together to promote overall well-being.

3. Prioritize Whole Foods

In a world where convenience often takes precedence, whole foods represent a return to the foundational essence of nutrition. They are foods that remain close to their natural state, unprocessed or minimally processed, retaining most of their nutrients and beneficial properties. Emphasizing whole foods in your diet is akin to selecting the raw, uncut gems in the realm of nutrition, as they offer a myriad of health advantages. Let's dive into the heart of this topic:

Why Whole Foods?

- **Nutrient Density:** Whole foods are packed with essential vitamins, minerals, fiber, and antioxidants. The absence of processing ensures that these nutrients are preserved in their most potent form.

- **Fewer Additives:** Processed foods often come with a slew of additives, preservatives, and artificial colors. By choosing whole foods, you sidestep many of these unwanted additives.

- **Support Digestive Health:** The fiber in whole foods, especially in whole grains, fruits, and vegetables, aids digestion, promotes regular bowel movements, and nurtures gut health.

- **Blood Sugar Control:** Whole foods, being rich in fiber and complex carbohydrates, help in slower sugar release, ensuring steady energy levels and reducing the risk of type 2 diabetes.

Key Whole Foods to Emphasize:

- **Whole Grains:** Unlike their refined counterparts, whole grains retain the bran, germ, and endosperm. This means you benefit from the full spectrum of their nutrients.

  - **Brown Rice:** A whole grain alternative to white rice, it's richer in fiber, vitamins, and minerals.

- **Quinoa:** A pseudo-grain, quinoa is a complete protein, offering all nine essential amino acids. It's also gluten-free and rich in various minerals.

- **Whole Wheat:** Opt for whole wheat bread or pasta instead of white versions. Whole wheat offers more fiber and a broader nutrient profile.

- **Oats:** An excellent source of soluble fiber, particularly beta-glucans, which are known for heart health benefits.

- **Fruits and Vegetables:** These are nature's multivitamins, offering a complex nutritional composition that supports various body functions.

  - **Daily Servings:** Strive for a minimum of five servings daily. This not only ensures adequate nutrient intake but also provides variety.

- **Colors Matter:** Different colored fruits and vegetables indicate varied nutrient profiles. For example, orange-colored ones like carrots are rich in beta-carotene, while dark greens like kale are high in iron and calcium.

Implementing Whole Foods in Your Diet:

1. **Start at the Store:** Make the outer aisles of the grocery store your primary shopping area since that's typically where fresh produce, grains, and proteins are found.

2. **Read Labels:** If a product has a long list of ingredients, especially ones hard to pronounce, it might be more processed. Aim for products with simpler, recognizable ingredient lists.

3. **Prepare Meals at Home:** Home cooking allows you to control ingredients and ensures you incorporate more whole foods.

4. **Limit Packaged Snacks:** Opt for fresh fruit, nuts, or yogurt as snacks over chips or cookies.

In conclusion, prioritizing whole foods is a transformative step toward embracing a nourishing, holistic diet. These nutrient powerhouses pave the path to improved overall health, energy, and vitality.

4. Limit Added Sugars and Salt

In the modern diet, added sugars and excessive salt have become pervasive and often concealed ingredients. They lurk in unexpected places, from bread to sauces to seemingly healthy snacks. While they might enhance flavor, their overconsumption poses health risks. Understanding and managing their intake is crucial for overall well-being. Let's explore this in depth:

The Concern with Added Sugars:

- **Health Implications:** Excessive sugar intake is linked to a multitude of health issues, including obesity, type 2 diabetes, heart disease, and even certain types of cancer. It can also lead to dental problems like cavities.

- **Hidden Sugars:** Sugars are often disguised under different names on ingredient lists, such as sucrose, high fructose corn syrup, barley malt, dextrose, maltose, and rice syrup, among others.

- **Natural Sweeteners:** While alternatives like honey, maple syrup, and agave nectar are more natural, they still add calories and can affect blood sugar. They do, however, offer some nutrients and antioxidants that refined sugars don't.

  - **Usage:** When using these sweeteners, moderation is key. While they're better than refined sugars, they should still be consumed sparingly.

The Issue with Excessive Salt:

- **Blood Pressure and Heart Health:** High sodium intake is associated with increased blood pressure, which can lead to heart disease and stroke. Salt makes the body retain water, increasing the strain on the heart and blood vessels.

- **Hidden Salt:** Packaged and processed foods, including seemingly healthy options, often contain more salt than you might expect. This includes items like bread, cereals, and canned goods.

- **Natural Flavor Enhancers:** Fortunately, there are countless ways to season your food without relying heavily on salt.

  - **Herbs:** Fresh or dried herbs like basil, rosemary, thyme, and cilantro can transform a dish.

  - **Spices:** Turmeric, cumin, paprika, and black pepper add flavor profiles from warm to spicy.

  - **Citrus and Vinegars:** A squeeze of lemon or a dash of balsamic vinegar can elevate a dish and reduce the need for salt.

Tips for Reducing Added Sugars and Salt:

1. **Become a Label Detective:** When shopping, make it a habit to check the nutritional facts and ingredient lists for sugars and sodium.

2. **Cook at Home:** Preparing meals from scratch gives you control over the ingredients, allowing you to limit added sugars and salt.

3. **Limit Sugary Drinks:** Beverages like sodas, energy drinks, and even some fruit juices can be significant sources of added sugars.

4. **Choose Unsweetened Snacks:** Opt for unsweetened or lightly sweetened yogurt, nut butters, and other snacks. If needed, you can add a small amount of a natural sweetener.

5. **Reduce Salt Gradually:** If you're used to salty foods, start by reducing the salt little by little, allowing your palate to adjust over time.

In conclusion, while sugars and salt naturally occur in many foods and are necessary for our body in moderation, it's the added amounts that we need to be wary of. By making conscious choices and savoring the natural flavors of whole foods, we can pave the path to a healthier, more balanced diet.

5. Include Healthy Fats

The narrative surrounding fats has experienced a significant shift over the past few decades. Once demonized and blamed for various health issues, we now understand that not all fats are created equal. In fact, healthy fats play vital roles in our bodies, supporting brain function, cell growth, and hormone production. Understanding which fats to embrace and which to limit or avoid can profoundly influence overall health. Let's break this down:

The Importance of Healthy Fats:

- **Brain Health:** The brain is composed of nearly 60% fat. Essential fatty acids, particularly omega-3s, are crucial for cognitive functions, memory, and mood regulation.

- **Vitamin Absorption:** Fats aid in the absorption of fat-soluble vitamins: A, D, E, and K.

- **Energy Source:** While carbohydrates are the body's primary energy source, fats serve as a sustained energy reserve.

- **Hormone Production:** Fats play a role in producing various hormones, including sex hormones like estrogen and testosterone.

Sources of Healthy Fats:

- **Avocados:** Rich in monounsaturated fats, avocados also offer fiber, potassium, and various antioxidants.

- **Olive Oil:** A staple in the Mediterranean diet, olive oil, especially extra virgin variety, is packed with heart-healthy monounsaturated fats and antioxidants.

- **Nuts:** Almonds, walnuts, cashews, and others provide a mix of monounsaturated and polyunsaturated fats, along with protein, fiber, and essential minerals.

- **Fatty Fish:** Salmon, mackerel, sardines, and trout are rich in omega-3 fatty acids, which have been linked to reduced inflammation and a lower risk of heart disease.

Fats to Limit or Avoid:

- **Saturated Fats:** Found mainly in animal products like butter, cheese, and red meat, saturated fats, when consumed in excess, can raise LDL (bad) cholesterol levels, increasing the risk of heart disease.

    - **Moderation is Key:** While it's wise to limit saturated fat intake, it doesn't need to be entirely eliminated. For instance, some studies suggest dairy fat may offer certain health benefits.

- **Trans Fats:** These are the real culprits to watch out for. Created by adding hydrogen to liquid vegetable oils to make them more solid, trans fats are linked to increased LDL cholesterol, reduced HDL (good) cholesterol, and a heightened risk of heart disease.

    - **Avoid Processed Foods:** Many baked goods, snacks, and fried foods can contain trans fats, even if the label says "0 grams of trans fats." Check for terms like "partially hydrogenated oils" in the ingredient list.

Incorporating Healthy Fats in Your Diet:

1. **Cook with Olive Oil:** Opt for olive oil over butter or margarine for cooking and salad dressings.

2. **Snack on Nuts:** A handful of mixed nuts can be a nutritious and satisfying snack, but be mindful of portions.

3. **Fatty Fish Twice a Week:** Aim to include fatty fish in your meals a couple of times per week for a dose of omega-3s.

4. **Avocado Toast:** A slice of whole-grain bread topped with avocado slices makes for a nutritious breakfast or snack.

5. **Check Labels:** Be vigilant about spotting trans fats in products. Remember, even if the nutritional info says "0g trans fats," it

could still contain up to 0.5 grams per serving.

In conclusion, healthy fats are indispensable to our well-being. By discerning the good from the not-so-good, and making informed choices, we not only nourish our bodies but also reap the numerous benefits that these essential nutrients bring to our overall health.

6. Stay Hydrated

Water is life – a statement that holds profound truth. Comprising around 60% of the human body, water plays a pivotal role in a plethora of physiological functions. From aiding digestion and nutrient absorption to temperature regulation and detoxification, staying adequately hydrated is paramount for overall health and well-being. Let's delve into the significance of hydration and strategies to ensure you're quenching your body's thirst optimally:

The Significance of Hydration:

- **Digestion and Nutrient Absorption:** Water assists in breaking down food in the stomach, facilitating nutrient absorption in the intestines.

- **Detoxification:** Through urine and sweat, water helps eliminate waste products and toxins from the body.

- **Temperature Regulation:** Sweating and its evaporation from the skin is a primary method by which the body cools down in hot conditions.

- **Joint Lubrication:** Water aids in keeping the cartilage around our joints hydrated and supple, ensuring smooth movement and reducing joint discomfort.

- **Skin Health:** Proper hydration can contribute to a radiant complexion, helping skin appear plump and youthful.

Hydration Guidelines:

- **8x8 Rule:** A common recommendation is the "8x8 rule," which suggests drinking eight 8-ounce glasses of water daily. However, this is a general guideline, and individual needs can vary.

- **Adjust Based on Activity:** If you're engaged in intense physical activity or sports, you'll need to increase your water intake. Sweating leads to fluid loss, which needs to be replenished.

- **Climate Considerations:** Living in or traveling to hotter climates or high altitudes can increase water requirements.

- **Listen to Your Body:** Thirst is an obvious signal to drink water. However, by the time you feel thirsty, you might already be mildly dehydrated. Regularly sipping on water throughout the day is a proactive approach.

Beverages to Limit or Monitor:

- **Sugary Drinks:** Beverages like sodas, sweet teas, and sugary fruit drinks can contribute to weight gain and other health issues. They can also cause rapid spikes and drops in blood sugar levels.

- **Caffeine:** While coffee and tea have their benefits, excessive caffeine can lead to dehydration, jitters, or sleep disturbances. Moderation is crucial, and ensuring you're drinking water alongside caffeinated beverages is wise.

- **Alcohol:** Alcohol acts as a diuretic, leading to increased urination and potential dehydration. If consuming alcohol, doing so in moderation and interspersing with water can help maintain hydration.

Hydration Tips:

1. **Flavor Your Water:** If plain water isn't enticing, try infusing it with slices of fruits, cucumbers, or herbs like mint for a refreshing twist.

2. **Hydration Foods:** Foods like watermelon, cucumbers, oranges, and strawberries have high water content and can contribute to your hydration.

3. **Set Reminders:** If you tend to forget to drink water, set reminders on your phone or use apps specifically designed to track your water intake.

4. **Carry a Reusable Water Bottle:** Keeping a water bottle on hand ensures that you can hydrate whenever the need arises.

In conclusion, understanding and respecting the body's need for water is fundamental for maintaining optimal health. Whether through pure water, hydrating foods, or other beverages, meeting your hydration needs is an investment in your well-being. Remember, every cell, tissue, and organ requires water to function correctly – it's truly the essence of life!

7. Consume Lean Proteins

Protein is often referred to as the building block of life. This macronutrient is fundamental for constructing and repairing tissues, making enzymes and hormones, and serving as a crucial energy source when carbohydrates are not available. While protein is abundant in various foods, it's essential to focus on lean, high-quality sources to ensure optimal health benefits. Let's dive into the world of lean proteins:

The Role of Proteins:

- **Tissue Repair and Growth:** Proteins are vital for building and repairing tissues, especially muscles, after exercises like strength training.

- **Enzymes and Hormones:** These biological catalysts and messengers in our body are often proteins, ensuring metabolic processes run smoothly.

- **Immune Response:** Antibodies, which help combat foreign invaders in the body, are proteins.

- **Energy Source:** In the absence of carbohydrates, proteins can be broken down to provide energy.

Sources of Lean Proteins:

- **Fish:** Especially fatty fish like salmon, mackerel, and sardines, which are not only excellent protein sources but also rich in heart-healthy omega-3 fatty acids.

- **Poultry:** Chicken and turkey breasts, when skinless, are lean sources of protein. They're versatile and can be prepared in various ways.

- **Tofu:** A plant-based protein derived from soybeans, tofu is a staple for many vegetarians and vegans. It's low in calories and can absorb flavors from the dishes it's cooked in.

- **Beans, Lentils, and Legumes:** These plant-based sources are not only rich in protein but also fiber, making them excellent for digestion and sustained energy. Examples include chickpeas, black beans, and green lentils.

Guidelines for Consuming Proteins:

- **Limit Red Meat:** While red meats like beef and lamb are rich in protein and other nutrients like iron and vitamin B12, they also contain higher levels of saturated fats. Frequent consumption has been linked to various health concerns, including heart diseases and certain cancers.

  - **Choose Wisely:** When consuming red meat, opt for lean cuts and consider grass-fed or organic varieties, which might have a better nutrient profile and fewer additives.

- **Diversify Your Protein Sources:** Just like other nutrients, it's essential to rotate your protein sources to ensure you're getting a range of associated nutrients. For example, fish provides omega-3s, while beans offer fiber.

- **Watch the Additives:** While focusing on the protein content, be mindful of additional components. For instance, processed meats like sausages or bacon often contain high levels of salt and preservatives.

Incorporating Lean Proteins in Your Diet:

1. **Stir-fries and Salads:** Both tofu and chicken can be easily added to vegetable stir-fries or salads for a protein boost.

2. **Protein-Packed Soups:** Lentil or chickpea soups are hearty, nutritious, and an excellent way to incorporate more protein.

3. **Grilled or Baked Fish:** Season fish fillets with herbs, lemon, and a touch of olive oil and grill or bake for a healthy protein-rich meal.

4. **Legume-Based Dishes:** Dishes like hummus (from chickpeas) or black bean tacos can be delicious ways to get your protein.

In conclusion, focusing on lean proteins ensures you're fueling your body with essential amino acids while limiting the intake of unwanted saturated fats and additives. With the myriad of available options, from plant-based to animal-derived, finding tasty and nutritious sources of protein has never been easier. Remember, balance and variety are keys to a holistic approach to consuming proteins.

8. Watch Portions

In today's era of supersized meals and gigantic food portions, portion control has become an increasingly important aspect of maintaining a healthy diet. Eating appropriate portions not only helps regulate calorie intake but also ensures a balanced consumption of nutrients. As the saying goes, too much of even a good thing can be bad. Let's explore the significance of portion control and ways to successfully manage it:

The Significance of Portion Control:

- **Calorie Management:** Controlling portions directly affects calorie intake. Overeating, even healthy foods, can lead to caloric surpluses, potentially resulting in weight gain.

- **Blood Sugar Regulation:** Consuming excessively large meals can lead to spikes and crashes in blood sugar, affecting energy levels and mood.

- **Digestive Health:** Overeating can strain the digestive system, leading to discomfort, bloating, or indigestion.

- **Satiety and Mindfulness:** Proper portion control aids in understanding satiety cues, enabling a more mindful eating experience.

Strategies for Effective Portion Control:

- **Use Smaller Plates:** This psychological trick makes portions appear larger. Filling a small plate gives a sense of abundance, while the same amount on a larger plate might seem insufficient.

- **Understand Serving Sizes:** Familiarize yourself with standard serving sizes. For instance, a serving of cooked meat is typically the size of a deck of cards, while a serving of cooked rice is roughly the size of a tennis ball.

- **Half-Plate Rule:** Aim to fill half of your plate with vegetables, a quarter with protein, and a quarter with grains or starches. This ensures a balanced meal while keeping portion sizes in check.

- **Limit Distractions:** Eating while watching TV, working, or browsing on a phone can lead to mindless eating and overconsumption. Focus on your meal to better recognize when you're satisfied.

- **Start with Less:** It's always possible to get seconds if you're still hungry, but starting with a smaller portion can help prevent unintentional overeating.

- **Stay Hydrated:** Drinking a glass of water before meals can help in feeling fuller faster.

- **Listen to Your Body:** Pay attention to hunger and fullness cues. It's okay to leave food on the plate if you feel satisfied.

Incorporating Portion Control in Daily Life:

1. **Pre-Portion Snacks:** Instead of eating directly from large packages, portion out

snacks into individual servings. This curbs the temptation to finish the entire bag.

2. **Avoid Eating Out of the Bag or Box:** Pouring a defined amount into a bowl can help prevent mindless munching.

3. **Split Restaurant Meals:** Restaurant portions can be notoriously large. Consider sharing a dish with someone or asking for half to be boxed up right away.

4. **Use Measuring Tools:** Especially when starting out, using measuring cups or a food scale can help in understanding what appropriate portion sizes look like.

In conclusion, while the quality of food is undeniably essential, the quantity should not be overlooked. Adopting effective portion control strategies can be a game-changer in one's journey to better health, weight management, and overall well-being. By cultivating mindfulness and staying informed about portion sizes, we can enjoy our meals to the fullest, both in terms of satisfaction and health benefits.

9. Limit Processed Foods

The modern food landscape is riddled with convenience – from microwave meals to canned soups and snack packs. While these processed foods might save time or satiate cravings, they often come at the expense of nutrition and overall health. Understanding the drawbacks of heavily processed foods and making informed dietary choices is paramount in today's age. Let's deep dive into why limiting processed foods is essential and how to navigate this challenge:

The Concerns with Processed Foods:

- **Nutrient Depletion:** Many processed foods have been stripped of their natural nutrients during manufacturing. Though some might be fortified afterward, they often lack the comprehensive nutrition of whole foods.

- **Additives & Preservatives:** Processed foods can be loaded with artificial colors, flavors, and preservatives, which may have questionable health impacts when consumed regularly.

- **High in Unhealthy Fats:** Many packaged foods contain trans fats or high levels of saturated fats, both of which are linked to increased heart disease risk.

- **Excessive Sugars:** Hidden sugars are ubiquitous in processed foods, from breakfast cereals to pasta sauces, leading to unintended high sugar intake.

- **Elevated Sodium Levels:** High salt content is common in processed foods, increasing the risk of hypertension and other cardiovascular issues.

- **Empty Calories:** Many processed foods offer calories without substantial nutritional value, leading to increased weight gain potential without satisfying hunger or nutrient needs.

Strategies to Limit Processed Foods:

- **Read Labels:** Acquaint yourself with ingredient lists and nutritional information. Look for foods with shorter ingredient lists and familiar components. Be wary of high sugar, sodium, and unhealthy fat contents.

- **Shop the Perimeter:** In many grocery stores, fresh produce, meats, and dairy are located along the perimeter, while processed foods dominate the inner aisles.

- **Cook at Home:** Preparing meals from scratch gives you control over ingredients, ensuring a fresh and nutritious meal.

- **Plan Ahead:** Meal planning and prepping can prevent last-minute reliance on processed foods when you're hungry or short on time.

- **Limit Sugary Beverages:** Sodas, energy drinks, and many fruit drinks are examples of highly processed beverages loaded with sugars and additives.

- **Educate Yourself:** Understand terms like "natural," "organic," and "fortified." Just because something claims to be natural doesn't mean it's not processed.

Alternatives to Processed Foods:

1. **Whole Grains vs. Refined:** Opt for whole grains like quinoa, brown rice, or whole grain bread over their refined counterparts.

2. **Fresh or Frozen Fruits & Veggies:** Instead of canned varieties, which might contain added sugars or salt, go for fresh or flash-frozen options.

3. **Homemade Snacks:** Instead of store-bought granola bars or chips, try making homemade alternatives using whole ingredients.

4. **Natural Sweeteners:** Use honey, maple syrup, or agave as sweeteners instead of high fructose corn syrup or artificial sweeteners.

5. **Whole Food Snacks:** Opt for snacks like nuts, seeds, or fresh fruits over candy bars or other processed snack foods.

In conclusion, while some level of food processing can be beneficial or benign (like frozen vegetables or canned beans), it's the heavily altered, additive-laden products that pose health concerns. Limiting such processed foods and emphasizing whole, fresh ingredients is a proactive approach towards better health, vitality, and longevity. With awareness and intention, we can navigate the modern food landscape wisely, making choices that nourish both our bodies and our souls.

10. Plan Ahead

In a world where fast food and microwaveable meals are always at our fingertips, it's easy to fall into the trap of convenience over health. The key to overcoming these temptations lies in a simple strategy: planning ahead. When we prepare for our meals and snacks in advance, we not only save time and money but also ensure that we're fueling our bodies with nutritious choices. Let's delve deeper into the concept of meal planning and prepping and how it can transform our eating habits:

The Benefits of Planning Ahead:

- **Nutritional Balance:** Planning allows for a comprehensive view of your meals, ensuring you're getting a balanced intake of proteins, fats, carbs, and micronutrients.

- **Cost-Efficient:** Buying in bulk and using ingredients in multiple meals often results in cost savings compared to frequent dining out or purchasing pre-made meals.

- **Time-Saving:** While it might require an initial time investment, having pre-prepared meals can save significant time on busy days.

- **Reduces Stress:** No more last-minute scrambles about what to eat. A plan provides clarity and peace of mind.

- **Minimizes Waste:** When meals are planned, grocery shopping becomes more purposeful, leading to less food waste.

Steps to Successful Meal Planning & Prepping:

1. **Assess Your Week:** Look at the week ahead. How many meals will you need? Are there days you know you'll be too busy to cook?

2. **Choose Your Meals:** Decide on a variety of meals to keep things interesting. Consider using some ingredients in multiple dishes to streamline shopping and preparation.

3. **Make a Shopping List:** Write down everything you'll need for your meals.

Organize the list by categories (produce, dairy, grains, etc.) to make the shopping trip efficient.

4. **Pick a Prep Day:** Dedicate a day (or two) for bulk preparation. This could mean chopping vegetables, marinating proteins, or fully cooking some meals.

5. **Storage Solutions:** Invest in quality storage containers. Labeling can also be beneficial, especially if you're freezing meals for later.

6. **Use Batch Cooking:** Make large portions of versatile foods (e.g., grilled chicken, quinoa, or roasted veggies) to use in different meals throughout the week.

7. **Consider Theme Nights:** Having a consistent theme, like "Taco Tuesday" or "Stir-Fry Friday," can simplify decision-making.

Tips for Staying on Track:

- **Keep It Flexible:** Life is unpredictable. If something comes up, adjust your plan. The key is to have nutritious options readily available.

- **Involve the Family:** Make it a group activity. When everyone is involved in choosing meals and prepping, there's more commitment to the plan.

- **Start Small:** If you're new to meal planning, begin with planning just a few days or specific meals like dinners. Gradually expand as you get the hang of it.

- **Utilize Technology:** There are numerous apps and websites dedicated to meal planning, complete with recipes and grocery lists.

- **Stay Inspired:** Regularly explore new recipes or cuisines to prevent monotony. Keeping your meals diverse ensures continued excitement and adherence to the plan.

In conclusion, planning ahead in terms of meals is a proactive approach to healthful eating. It reduces the dependency on less nutritious, convenience-based options, setting you up for success in your health journey. By dedicating some time and thought to your food in advance, you're prioritizing not only your health but also the quality and enjoyment of what you eat. Embrace the process, enjoy the creativity, and relish the rewards of your well-laid plans!

11. Listen to Your Body

The essence of intuitive eating lies in the simplicity of this statement: "Listen to your body." While this sounds straightforward, modern life—with its abundance of food marketing, diet culture, and societal pressures—often drowns out our body's innate signals. Yet, by tuning into our internal cues, we can cultivate a healthier, more harmonious relationship with food. Let's delve into the importance of listening to our bodies and how to cultivate this essential skill.

Why Listening to Your Body Matters:

- **Natural Regulation:** Our bodies have built-in mechanisms to signal hunger and fullness, helping regulate energy intake.

- **Prevents Overeating:** Paying attention to satiety cues can prevent consuming more than our body needs, which can lead to weight gain and discomfort.

- **Enhances Enjoyment:** By eating when truly hungry, food tastes better, and the experience is more satisfying.

- **Reduces Stress:** Removing the external rules and restrictions about when and what to eat can reduce anxiety around meals.

- **Promotes Self-awareness:** Recognizing and understanding our body's cues can foster a deeper connection with ourselves.

Navigating Hunger vs. Emotional Eating:

1. **True Hunger:** This is a physiological need for food. Signs might include a rumbling stomach, low energy, irritability, or difficulty concentrating. It comes on gradually and can be satisfied with any food.

2. **Emotional Eating:** This stems from feelings rather than physical hunger. You might crave specific comfort foods and feel the urge to eat suddenly, even after a recent

meal. It's often tied to emotions like stress, boredom, sadness, or even joy.

Strategies to Listen to Your Body:

- **Mindful Eating:** This involves being fully present during meals. Turn off distractions like TV or smartphones. Focus on the flavors, textures, and sensations of eating. This heightened awareness can help you better detect satiety cues.

- **Slow Down:** It takes time for the brain to recognize that the stomach is full. Taking your time, chewing thoroughly, and pausing between bites can give your body the time it needs to signal fullness.

- **Check-in Regularly:** Periodically ask yourself how hungry or full you are. This can prevent mindless eating and make you more attuned to your body's signals.

- **Understand Your Triggers:** If you find yourself reaching for food when not hungry, consider what might be triggering this desire. Is it stress? Boredom? Social pressures? Recognizing these can help address the root cause rather than using food as a band-aid.

- **Stay Hydrated:** Thirst can sometimes be mistaken for hunger. If you feel hungry shortly after eating, consider having a glass of water and waiting a bit to see if the sensation passes.

- **Seek Support:** If emotional eating is a consistent challenge, consider seeking support. This could be through therapy, support groups, or nutrition counseling.

Incorporating Intuitive Eating Principles:

1. **Reject Diet Mentality:** Avoid restrictive diets that impose strict rules and can warp your relationship with food.

2. **Honor Your Hunger:** Eat when hungry. This prevents excessive hunger that can lead to overeating later.

3. **Feel Your Fullness:** Recognize when you're comfortably full and give yourself permission to stop eating.

4. **Address Emotions Without Food:** Find other ways to cope with emotions— whether it's through movement, journaling, talking to someone, or practicing relaxation techniques.

In conclusion, listening to our body is a journey back to basics—a reconnection with the innate wisdom we were born with. By honoring our hunger and fullness, understanding the difference between physiological and emotional eating, and practicing mindfulness, we can foster a balanced, joyful, and healthful relationship with food. This approach champions self-care, compassion, and the understanding that our bodies are wise—if only we take the time to listen.

12. Limit Alcohol Intake

In a world that often celebrates and socializes over drinks, understanding the role of alcohol in a healthy lifestyle is paramount. While some studies suggest certain benefits from moderate alcohol consumption, especially from drinks like red wine, it's crucial to balance these benefits against potential drawbacks. Learning to consume alcohol mindfully and in moderation can lead to a more balanced and health-conscious approach to drinking. Let's dive deeper into why and how to limit alcohol intake.

Why Limiting Alcohol Matters:

- **Caloric Intake:** Alcohol contains 7 calories per gram, making it calorie-dense. Drinking can quickly add extra, empty calories to your daily intake, potentially leading to weight gain.

- **Nutritional Impact:** Alcohol can interfere with the absorption of essential nutrients, including vitamins and minerals.

- **Mental Health:** Excessive alcohol consumption can exacerbate symptoms of depression, anxiety, and other mental health issues.

- **Liver Health:** Chronic heavy drinking can lead to various liver problems, including fatty liver, hepatitis, fibrosis, and cirrhosis.

- **Increased Risk:** High alcohol consumption is linked to an elevated risk of several cancers, cardiovascular diseases, and other health problems.

- **Impaired Judgment:** Alcohol affects the central nervous system and can lead to reduced reaction times, poor decision-making, and riskier behaviors.

Navigating Moderate Drinking:

1. **Understand Moderation:** For many, moderate drinking is defined as up to one drink per day for women and up to two drinks per day for men.

2. **Recognize a Standard Drink:** This typically
   means 14 grams (0.6 ounces) of pure
   alcohol—roughly equivalent to 5 ounces of
   wine, 12 ounces of beer, or 1.5 ounces of
   distilled spirits.

3. **Choose Healthier Options:** Some drinks
   have added health benefits. For example,
   red wine contains resveratrol, which may
   offer heart health benefits. However, it's
   essential to weigh these benefits against
   potential risks.

Strategies to Limit Alcohol Intake:

- **Mindful Drinking:** Before reaching for a
  drink, consider why you're choosing to
  consume alcohol. Is it out of habit, social
  pressure, or a genuine desire? Becoming
  more intentional can help reduce
  unnecessary drinking.

- **Alternate with Water:** For every alcoholic
  drink you have, consume a glass of water.
  This can help with hydration, reduce the

overall amount of alcohol consumed, and pace your drinking.

- **Eat Beforehand:** Consuming alcohol on an empty stomach can lead to faster intoxication. Eating a balanced meal before drinking can slow alcohol absorption.

- **Set Limits:** Decide in advance how many drinks you'll have and stick to it. This pre-set boundary can help prevent overindulgence.

- **Avoid Drinking as a Coping Mechanism:** If you find yourself reaching for alcohol to deal with stress, sadness, or other emotions, seek healthier coping strategies or consider professional support.

- **Partake in Alcohol-Free Days:** Dedicate certain days of the week to be alcohol-free. This can break the habit of daily drinking and reduce overall consumption.

- **Educate Yourself:** The more you understand about alcohol's effects on the body, the more empowered you'll be to make informed decisions.

Making Healthier Alcohol Choices:

1. **Opt for Red Wine:** As mentioned, red wine contains compounds like resveratrol that may have heart-protective benefits.

2. **Avoid Sugary Mixers:** If you're having a mixed drink, be wary of sugary sodas, juices, or premade mixes. Opt for seltzer or a splash of fresh juice.

3. **Consider Lower-Alcohol Options:** Some beers and wines have lower alcohol content, allowing you to enjoy a drink without consuming as much alcohol.

In conclusion, alcohol can be part of a balanced lifestyle when consumed mindfully and in moderation. Recognizing its potential impact on health and well-being, setting boundaries, and making informed choices can allow you to enjoy the social aspects of drinking without compromising your health. Remember, it's always okay to abstain, and seeking the middle ground ensures that you prioritize your well-being in every sip.

13. Stay Active

Physical activity, often intertwined with the concept of a balanced diet, plays a pivotal role in holistic health and well-being. Just as a car requires fuel to function, our bodies need regular movement to operate at their best. Incorporating a consistent exercise routine can enhance both mental and physical health, complementing the benefits of a nutritious diet. Let's dive deep into the importance of staying active and the multitude of benefits it offers.

Why Staying Active Matters:

- **Cardiovascular Health:** Regular physical activity strengthens the heart and improves circulation, reducing the risk of cardiovascular diseases such as hypertension, heart disease, and stroke.

- **Bone and Muscle Strength:** Weight-bearing exercises can increase bone density, decreasing the risk of osteoporosis. Meanwhile, strength training helps maintain and build muscle mass.

- **Weight Management:** Physical activity helps burn calories, aiding in weight control and complementing a balanced diet.

- **Mental Health and Mood:** Exercise releases endorphins—natural mood lifters. This can help alleviate symptoms of depression, anxiety, and stress.

- **Improved Sleep:** Regular physical activity can lead to better sleep quality and increased energy during the day.

- **Metabolic Health:** Exercise can help regulate blood sugar levels and increase insulin sensitivity, reducing the risk of type 2 diabetes.

- **Enhanced Immunity:** Moderate, consistent exercise can bolster the immune system, potentially reducing the risk of chronic diseases and infections.

Finding the Right Physical Activity:

1. **Aerobic Activities:** These are endurance-building exercises that elevate heart rate. Examples include walking, jogging, swimming, and cycling.

2. **Strength Training:** Focused on building muscle mass. This includes weight lifting, resistance band exercises, and bodyweight exercises like push-ups and squats.

3. **Flexibility and Balance:** Activities like yoga and tai chi enhance flexibility, balance, and muscle tone, which is especially beneficial as we age.

4. **Functional Fitness:** This focuses on training the body for the activities performed in daily life, such as squatting, reaching, or lifting.

Strategies to Stay Active:

- **Consistency is Key:** It's better to engage in moderate activity regularly than to have intense workouts sporadically. Aim for at least 150 minutes of moderate-intensity aerobic activity each week.

- **Mix It Up:** Diverse workouts can prevent monotony and engage different muscle groups. Rotate between aerobic exercises, strength training, and flexibility exercises.

- **Set Goals:** Whether it's to run a certain distance, lift a particular weight, or achieve a fitness milestone, goals provide motivation and a sense of purpose.

- **Find a Buddy:** Having a workout partner can be motivating, making exercise sessions enjoyable and providing accountability.

- **Listen to Your Body:** While it's important to challenge oneself, it's equally critical to recognize when to rest. Overtraining can lead to injuries.

- **Incorporate Movement into Daily Life:** Opt for stairs instead of elevators, park further from entrances, or consider walking or cycling for short errands.

- **Stay Motivated:** Whether it's through music, tracking apps, or joining a local fitness group, find what drives you and stick to it.

Complementing Diet with Physical Activity:

1. **Fuel Up Right:** Consume a balanced meal or snack 1-2 hours before exercising. This provides the necessary energy for your workout.

2. **Stay Hydrated:** Drink water before, during, and after workouts to stay hydrated.

3. **Recover Properly:** Post-exercise, consume a mix of proteins and carbs to repair muscles and replenish glycogen stores.

In conclusion, staying active is an integral pillar of a healthy lifestyle, harmonizing with a nutritious diet to optimize overall well-being.

From cardiovascular benefits to improved mental health, the perks of consistent movement are manifold. As you journey through a life of healthful eating, remember that every step, jog, or stretch you take echoes the commitment to nourishing your body, mind, and soul.

14. Consult a Nutritionist or Dietitian

In our journey to better health and well-being, expert advice can often be the compass that guides us in the right direction. While there's a plethora of information available on nutrition, not all of it may be applicable or beneficial to everyone. Our bodies, lifestyles, and health conditions are unique, requiring tailored strategies for optimal results. This is where consulting a nutritionist or dietitian becomes invaluable. Let's delve into why seeking professional counsel is essential and how it can shape our health trajectories.

Why Consulting a Professional Matters:

- **Individualized Approach:** Generic dietary advice may not account for individual health conditions, allergies, intolerances, or preferences. A nutritionist or dietitian can tailor recommendations to your specific needs.

- **Evidence-Based Advice:** Registered dietitians and nutritionists base their advice on scientific evidence and their extensive training, ensuring recommendations are sound and up-to-date.

- **Addressing Health Concerns:** For individuals with specific health conditions like diabetes, heart disease, gastrointestinal disorders, or obesity, personalized dietary plans can make a substantial difference in managing and potentially improving these conditions.

- **Optimizing Nutrient Intake:** A professional can help ensure that you're getting all the essential nutrients in the right amounts, especially if you have dietary restrictions.

- **Behavioral Strategies:** Beyond just knowing what to eat, professionals can provide strategies to help you change eating behaviors, overcome challenges, and maintain a healthy lifestyle long term.

Navigating the Consultation Process:

1. **Initial Assessment:** The first meeting usually involves a detailed discussion about your current eating habits, health concerns, lifestyle, and dietary preferences.

2. **Goal Setting:** Together, you'll outline specific, achievable nutrition and health goals based on your individual needs and circumstances.

3. **Customized Plan:** The nutritionist or dietitian will provide a tailored eating plan, considering factors like your age, activity level, health conditions, and dietary preferences.

4. **Ongoing Support:** Regular follow-up sessions can help track progress, address challenges, and refine your dietary plan as necessary.

Things to Consider When Consulting:

- **Credentials Matter:** Ensure that the professional you consult is credentialed. In many countries, 'dietitian' is a regulated term, while 'nutritionist' may not be. Check their qualifications and any associated professional affiliations.

- **Open Communication:** Be honest about your habits, challenges, and preferences. The more information you provide, the better the advice will be tailored to your needs.

- **Stay Proactive:** While a professional provides guidance, the onus of implementation lies with you. Engage actively in the process, ask questions, and seek clarity when needed.

- **Embrace Flexibility:** Nutritional needs and personal circumstances can change. It's essential to be adaptable and revisit your plan as required.

- **Consider Costs:** Consulting fees can vary. Some insurance plans may cover nutrition counseling, especially if it's for a specific medical condition. It's wise to check in advance.

Complementary Role in Overall Health:

1. **Working with Other Healthcare Professionals:** Often, dietitians and nutritionists collaborate with doctors, physical therapists, and other healthcare providers to offer comprehensive care.

2. **Holistic Approach:** Beyond just food, many professionals also consider factors like sleep, stress, physical activity, and mental well-being when providing advice.

In conclusion, while the journey to optimal health may start with personal choices and determination, consulting experts like nutritionists and dietitians can offer the roadmap to navigate it more effectively. These professionals provide a wealth of knowledge, tailored strategies, and support, ensuring that your nutrition choices align with your unique body and health goals. Remember, investing in expert advice is an investment in long-term well-being, making every bite a step closer to a healthier you.

15. Stay Educated

In the age of information, nutritional advice can be found at every corner—be it in the form of articles, blogs, videos, or social media posts. However, not all information is created equal. Nutritional science, like all sciences, is a dynamic field. New research and discoveries constantly reshape our understanding of what's best for our bodies. The onus, therefore, is on us to sift through the noise and ensure our decisions are informed and rational. Let's discuss the importance of staying educated in nutrition and the best strategies to achieve it.

The Imperative of Continued Education in Nutrition:

- **Navigating Changing Paradigms:** What was once considered nutritional gospel may be debunked or modified as new research emerges. Regular education keeps you aligned with the most current, scientifically-backed guidance.

- **Making Informed Decisions:** Knowledge empowers. Being educated means you're better equipped to make decisions about what goes into your body, ensuring your dietary choices serve your health goals.

- **Avoiding Fads and Myths:** The world of nutrition is rife with fleeting trends and myths. A solid foundation of knowledge helps you discern fact from fiction.

- **Advocating for Your Health:** The more you know, the better you can advocate for your health, whether it's in discussions with healthcare professionals, making grocery choices, or when dining out.

Strategies to Stay Updated:

1. **Reputable Sources:** Seek information from credible sources like scientific journals, government health websites, or established health organizations. Examples include the World Health Organization, the National Institutes of

Health, or the Academy of Nutrition and Dietetics.

2. **Continuous Learning:** Consider enrolling in nutrition courses, attending workshops, or participating in webinars. Even basic courses can significantly enhance your understanding.

3. **Consult Experts:** Engage with dietitians, nutritionists, or medical professionals. They often have access to the latest research and can offer evidence-based advice.

4. **Read Widely but Critically:** While it's essential to read widely, it's equally important to approach information with a critical mindset. Check for references, the credibility of the author, and be wary of sources that make grandiose, unsupported claims.

5. **Stay Away from Extreme Views:** Extremist views, whether for or against a particular diet or nutrient, often lack a balanced

perspective. Nutrition is multifaceted, and what works for one person might not work for another.

6. **Engage with Scientific Literature:** Platforms like Google Scholar or PubMed provide access to a wealth of scientific studies. While they can be technical, reading abstracts or summaries can give you an idea of current research directions.

Avoiding Pitfalls:

- **Beware of Confirmation Bias:** We often seek information that confirms our pre-existing beliefs. Challenge yourself to understand opposing viewpoints and weigh the evidence before forming an opinion.

- **Steer Clear of Celebrity Endorsements:** Just because a celebrity endorses a diet or product doesn't mean it's scientifically valid or suitable for everyone.

- **Watch Out for Sales Pitches:** Be cautious of sources that push a particular product,

diet, or supplement as a 'miracle solution'.
True nutrition advice is usually more
nuanced.

Embracing a Holistic View:

1. **Integrate New Knowledge:** As you learn,
   find ways to incorporate this knowledge
   into your daily life, making necessary
   adjustments to your diet and lifestyle.

2. **Share What You Learn:** Sharing knowledge
   can not only help others but also reinforce
   your understanding.

In conclusion, the journey to optimal nutrition
is as much about what you eat as it is about
understanding why you eat it. Staying educated
ensures that your dietary choices are grounded
in science and rationality. It's a proactive
approach, acknowledging that your health is an
investment and that knowledge is one of the
most potent tools in your arsenal. In a world
overflowing with nutritional advice, let
education be your compass, guiding you
towards choices that truly nourish.

Final Thoughts

Nutrition, like life itself, is about balance. It's a dance between indulgence and discipline, between listening to our bodies and adhering to the wisdom of science. As we navigate the vast landscape of nutritional information, it's essential to remember that perfection isn't the goal. Instead, it's the pursuit of a sustainable, joyful, and healthful relationship with food. Let's take a moment to reflect on this journey and the essence of what it truly means to eat healthily.

The Beauty of Occasional Indulgence:

- **A Slice of Life:** Every culture celebrates with food, be it birthdays, weddings, or festivals. These occasions often involve dishes that aren't necessarily 'healthy' but are rich in tradition, taste, and joy. Allowing ourselves to partake in these moments adds depth to our life experiences.

- **Reset and Recharge:** Sometimes, a sweet treat or a hearty meal serves as comfort, providing a mental break from routine. It's a reminder that food isn't just fuel; it's also pleasure.

- **Avoiding the Deprivation Mindset:** Constantly denying ourselves can lead to feelings of deprivation, which can eventually trigger overindulgence or binge eating. Occasional treats can prevent this cycle by offering a healthy release.

Balance: The Golden Key:

- **The 80/20 Rule:** A popular guideline suggests that if you eat healthily 80% of the time, it's okay to indulge in less-healthy choices the remaining 20%. This perspective promotes balance and adaptability.

- **Nutritional Equilibrium:** Balance isn't just about when we indulge but also about ensuring our overall diet comprises varied nutrients. For instance, if one meal is carb-heavy, perhaps the next can be rich in proteins and veggies.

- **Mental and Emotional Balance:** Eating should also be about nurturing our mental and emotional well-being. Sometimes, the healthiest choice for our minds might be that slice of chocolate cake or those comfort foods that evoke cherished memories.

Consistency Over Perfection:

- **Habits Over Diets:** Long-term health isn't defined by the occasional dessert or fried meal; it's about the habits we cultivate over time. A consistent pattern of nutritious eating will always outweigh the occasional divergence.

- **Progress, Not Perfection:** Every meal is an opportunity. If you make a choice you regret, don't despair. The next meal offers a fresh start. Celebrate the progress you make, rather than aiming for unattainable perfection.

The Joyful Journey of Eating:

- **Rediscover Flavors:** Healthy foods aren't just about greens and grains. They encompass a vast array of flavors, from the tang of berries to the umami of mushrooms. Revel in this culinary adventure.

- **Be Present:** Whether you're indulging or eating a simple salad, be present. Savor every bite, relish the textures, and appreciate the nourishment you're providing your body.

- **Learning and Adapting:** As we've discussed throughout, staying educated is crucial. But it's not just about acquiring knowledge—it's about adapting, evolving, and learning from our bodies and experiences.

In wrapping up, it's essential to remember that the heart of healthy eating isn't restriction—it's respect. Respect for our bodies, our traditions, and the vast tapestry of foods that nature offers. Every bite, be it a carefully crafted salad or a decadent piece of cake, tells a story. As you journey through the world of nutrition, write your story with joy, balance, and consistency, knowing that every chapter is a step towards a vibrant, healthful life. Embrace the journey, for in the realm of nutrition, the journey itself is the true feast.

Delicious Healthy Recipes

1. Quinoa and Black Bean Salad

Servings: 4

Ingredients:

- 1 cup cooked quinoa
- 1 can (15 oz) black beans, rinsed and drained
- 1 red bell pepper, diced
- 1/2 cup fresh cilantro, chopped
- 2 limes, juiced
- 2 tbsp olive oil
- Salt and pepper to taste

Instructions:

1. Mix all ingredients in a large bowl.
2. Refrigerate for an hour before serving.

Nutrition Facts (per serving = approx. 1 cup):

- Calories: 220
- Protein: 9g
- Carbohydrates: 35g
- Fat: 7g
- Fiber: 8g
- Sugar: 2g

2. Spinach and Feta Stuffed Chicken

Servings: 4

Ingredients:

- 4 chicken breasts
- 1 cup spinach, cooked and drained
- 1/2 cup feta cheese
- 1 tsp olive oil
- Salt and pepper

Instructions:

1. Preheat oven to 375°F (190°C).
2. Slice a pocket into each chicken breast and stuff with spinach and feta.
3. Seal with toothpicks.
4. Brush each breast with olive oil and season with salt and pepper.
5. Bake for about 25-30 minutes or until chicken is cooked through.

Nutrition Facts (per serving = 1 stuffed chicken breast):

- Calories: 285
- Protein: 28g
- Carbohydrates: 2g
- Fat: 18g
- Fiber: 1g
- Sugar: 1g

3. Chickpea and Vegetable Stir-fry

Servings: 4

Ingredients:

- 2 cups cooked chickpeas
- 2 bell peppers, sliced
- 1 cup broccoli florets
- 1 carrot, sliced
- 2 tbsp soy sauce
- 1 tbsp sesame oil

Instructions:

1. Heat sesame oil in a pan.
2. Add the vegetables and stir-fry for 5 minutes.
3. Add chickpeas and soy sauce and cook for another 5 minutes.

Nutrition Facts (per serving = approx. 1 cup):

- Calories: 215
- Protein: 8g
- Carbohydrates: 31g
- Fat: 7g
- Fiber: 8g
- Sugar: 6g

4. Berry Yogurt Parfait

Servings: 2

Ingredients:

- 2 cups Greek yogurt

- 1 cup mixed berries (blueberries, raspberries, strawberries)

- 2 tbsp honey

- 2 tbsp granola

Instructions:

1. In a glass, layer yogurt, berries, and granola.

2. Drizzle honey on top.

Nutrition Facts (per serving):

- Calories: 230

- Protein: 15g

- Carbohydrates: 35g

- Fat: 2g

- Fiber: 2g

- Sugar: 28g

5. Sweet Potato Soup

Servings: 4

Ingredients:

- 2 sweet potatoes, peeled and diced
- 4 cups vegetable broth
- 1 onion, diced
- 2 garlic cloves, minced
- 1 tbsp olive oil
- Salt and pepper to taste

Instructions:

1. In a pot, heat olive oil and sauté onions and garlic.
2. Add sweet potatoes and vegetable broth.
3. Simmer until sweet potatoes are tender.
4. Blend until smooth. Season with salt and pepper.

Nutrition Facts (per serving = approx. 1 cup):

- Calories: 155
- Protein: 3g
- Carbohydrates: 35g
- Fat: 2g
- Fiber: 5g
- Sugar: 8g

6. Zucchini Noodles with Pesto

Servings: 4

Ingredients:

- 4 zucchinis, spiralized

- 1/2 cup pesto

- 1/4 cup grated Parmesan

Instructions:

1. Toss zucchini noodles with pesto.

2. Top with grated Parmesan before serving.

Nutrition Facts (per serving = approx. 1 cup):

- Calories: 180

- Protein: 6g

- Carbohydrates: 6g

- Fat: 15g

- Fiber: 1g

- Sugar: 4g

7. Lentil Salad

Servings: 4

Ingredients:

- 2 cups cooked green lentils
- 1 tomato, diced
- 1 cucumber, diced
- 1/4 cup feta cheese, crumbled
- 2 tbsp olive oil
- 2 tbsp lemon juice
- Salt and pepper to taste

Instructions:

1. Mix all ingredients in a bowl.

Nutrition Facts (per serving = approx. 1 cup):

- Calories: 260
- Protein: 13g
- Carbohydrates: 30g
- Fat: 10g
- Fiber: 15g
- Sugar: 4g

8. Oatmeal with Almonds and Berries

Servings: 2

Ingredients:

- 1 cup rolled oats

- 2 cups almond milk

- 1/2 cup mixed berries

- 1/4 cup almonds, chopped

- 1 tbsp honey

Instructions:

1. Cook oats in almond milk until soft.

2. Top with berries, almonds, and drizzle with honey.

Nutrition Facts (per serving):

- Calories: 280

- Protein: 8g

- Carbohydrates: 38g

- Fat: 11g

- Fiber: 7g

- Sugar: 13g

9. Grilled Salmon with Asparagus

Servings: 4

Ingredients:

- 4 salmon fillets
- 1 bunch asparagus, trimmed
- 2 tbsp olive oil
- Salt and pepper to taste
- Lemon wedges for serving

Instructions:

1. Season salmon and asparagus with olive oil, salt, and pepper.
2. Grill until salmon is cooked and asparagus is tender.
3. Serve with lemon wedges.

Nutrition Facts (per serving = 1 fillet and approx. 5 asparagus spears):

- Calories: 345
- Protein: 35g
- Carbohydrates: 2g
- Fat: 22g
- Fiber: 1g
- Sugar: 1g

10. Cauliflower Rice Stir-fry

Servings: 4

Ingredients:

- 1 head of cauliflower, riced
- 1 bell pepper, sliced
- 1 carrot, sliced
- 2 eggs, scrambled
- 2 tbsp soy sauce
- 1 tbsp sesame oil

Instructions:

1. Heat sesame oil in a pan.
2. Add vegetables and stir-fry for 5 minutes.
3. Push veggies to the side, scramble eggs in the pan.
4. Add cauliflower rice and soy sauce. Cook for another 5-7 minutes.

Nutrition Facts (per serving = approx. 1 cup):

- Calories: 145
- Protein: 7g
- Carbohydrates: 15g
- Fat: 7g
- Fiber: 5g
- Sugar: 5g

11. Lemon Herb Grilled Chicken

Servings: 4

Ingredients:

- 4 chicken breasts

- 2 lemons, juiced

- 2 tbsp olive oil

- 1 tbsp chopped fresh herbs (rosemary, thyme, parsley)

- Salt and pepper

Instructions:

1. Marinate chicken in lemon juice, olive oil, herbs, salt, and pepper for at least 30 minutes.

2. Grill until fully cooked.

Nutrition Facts (per serving = 1 chicken breast):

- Calories: 265

- Protein: 28g

- Carbohydrates: 3g

- Fat: 15g

- Fiber: 0g

- Sugar: 1g

12. Beef and Broccoli Stir-fry

Servings: 4

Ingredients:

- 500g beef slices
- 2 cups broccoli florets
- 3 tbsp soy sauce
- 2 tbsp oyster sauce
- 1 tbsp sesame oil
- 2 garlic cloves, minced

Instructions:

1. In a pan, heat sesame oil and sauté garlic.
2. Add beef and cook until browned.
3. Add broccoli, soy sauce, and oyster sauce. Stir-fry until broccoli is tender.

Nutrition Facts (per serving):

- Calories: 320
- Protein: 30g
- Carbohydrates: 10g
- Fat: 18g
- Fiber: 2g
- Sugar: 3g

13. Turkey and Avocado Wraps

Servings: 4

Ingredients:

- 4 whole-grain tortillas
- 500g sliced turkey breast
- 2 avocados, sliced
- 1 tomato, sliced
- Lettuce

Instructions:

1. Lay out tortilla. Layer turkey, avocado slices, tomato, and lettuce.
2. Roll up and serve.

Nutrition Facts (per serving = 1 wrap):

- Calories: 340
- Protein: 25g
- Carbohydrates: 35g
- Fat: 13g
- Fiber: 6g
- Sugar: 4g

14. Pork Chops with Apple Sauce

Servings: 4

Ingredients:

- 4 pork chops
- 2 apples, peeled, cored, and chopped
- 1 tbsp honey
- 1/2 tsp cinnamon
- Salt and pepper

Instructions:

1. Season pork chops with salt and pepper. Grill or pan-fry until cooked.
2. In a saucepan, cook apples until soft. Mash and mix in honey and cinnamon.
3. Serve pork chops with a dollop of apple sauce.

Nutrition Facts (per serving = 1 pork chop with sauce):

- Calories: 340
- Protein: 30g
- Carbohydrates: 15g
- Fat: 18g
- Fiber: 2g
- Sugar: 12g

15. Spaghetti Squash and Meatballs

Servings: 4

Ingredients:

- 1 spaghetti squash, halved and seeds removed
- 500g lean ground beef
- 1 can crushed tomatoes
- 1 onion, chopped
- 2 garlic cloves, minced
- 1 tbsp olive oil
- Salt, pepper, and Italian herbs

Instructions:

1. Bake spaghetti squash at 375°F (190°C) for 45 minutes.
2. In a bowl, mix beef, salt, pepper, and herbs. Form into meatballs.
3. In a pan, heat olive oil. Sauté onions and garlic. Add meatballs and brown them.
4. Add crushed tomatoes and simmer until meatballs are cooked.
5. Scrape the inside of the spaghetti squash to create "noodles". Serve with meatballs and sauce.

Nutrition Facts (per serving):

- Calories: 380

- Protein: 28g

- Carbohydrates: 30g

- Fat: 18g

- Fiber: 6g

- Sugar: 12g

16. Grilled Lamb with Mint Sauce

Servings: 4

Ingredients:

- 4 lamb steaks
- 2 tbsp olive oil
- Salt and pepper
- 1/2 cup fresh mint, chopped
- 1 tbsp vinegar
- 1 tbsp honey

Instructions:

1. Season lamb with olive oil, salt, and pepper. Grill until preferred doneness.
2. Mix mint, vinegar, and honey for the sauce.
3. Serve lamb with mint sauce drizzled on top.

Nutrition Facts (per serving = 1 lamb steak with sauce):

- Calories: 370
- Protein: 28g
- Carbohydrates: 8g
- Fat: 25g
- Fiber: 0g
- Sugar: 7g

17. Shrimp and Garlic Zoodles

Servings: 4

Ingredients:

- 500g shrimp, peeled and deveined
- 4 zucchinis, spiralized
- 4 garlic cloves, minced
- 2 tbsp olive oil
- Salt and pepper
- Chili flakes (optional)

Instructions:

1. In a pan, heat olive oil. Sauté garlic until fragrant.
2. Add shrimp and cook until pink.
3. Add zoodles and cook for 2-3 minutes. Season with salt, pepper, and chili flakes.

Nutrition Facts (per serving):

- Calories: 230
- Protein: 25g
- Carbohydrates: 10g
- Fat: 10g
- Fiber: 2g
- Sugar: 5g

18. Chicken Caesar Salad

Servings: 4

Ingredients:

- 4 chicken breasts
- 2 heads romaine lettuce, chopped
- 1/2 cup grated Parmesan
- Caesar dressing (preferably low-fat)
- Croutons

Instructions:

1. Grill chicken breasts and slice them.
2. In a bowl, toss lettuce, Parmesan, dressing, and croutons. Top with chicken slices.

Nutrition Facts (per serving):

- Calories: 310
- Protein: 30g
- Carbohydrates: 12g
- Fat: 16g
- Fiber: 2g
- Sugar: 3g

19. Beef and Quinoa Stuffed Peppers

Servings: 4

Ingredients:

- 4 bell peppers, tops removed and deseeded
- 500g lean ground beef
- 1 cup cooked quinoa
- 1 can crushed tomatoes
- 1 onion, chopped
- 2 garlic cloves, minced
- 1 tbsp olive oil
- Salt, pepper, and herbs

Instructions:

1. In a pan, heat olive oil. Sauté onions and garlic.
2. Add beef and cook until browned. Mix in quinoa and crushed tomatoes. Season.
3. Stuff peppers with the mixture. Bake at 375°F (190°C) for 25-30 minutes.

Nutrition Facts (per serving = 1 stuffed pepper):

- Calories: 370
- Protein: 30g
- Carbohydrates: 30g

- Fat: 15g

- Fiber: 5g

- Sugar: 10g

20. Chicken and Vegetable Kabobs

Servings: 4

Ingredients:

- 4 chicken breasts, cubed
- 2 bell peppers, cubed
- 1 zucchini, sliced
- 1 red onion, cubed
- Olive oil
- Salt, pepper, and herbs

Instructions:

1. Skewer chicken and vegetables alternately.
2. Brush with olive oil and season.
3. Grill until chicken is fully cooked.

Nutrition Facts (per serving = 2 kabobs):

- Calories: 260
- Protein: 28g
- Carbohydrates: 10g
- Fat: 12g
- Fiber: 2g
- Sugar: 5g

21. Pork and Pineapple Tacos

Servings: 4

Ingredients:

- 500g pork tenderloin, sliced

- 8 small corn tortillas

- 1 cup pineapple, diced

- 1 red onion, chopped

- 1 jalapeño, minced

- 1 lime, juiced

- Salt and pepper

Instructions:

1. Cook pork slices until fully cooked.

2. Mix pineapple, red onion, jalapeño, lime juice, salt, and pepper for salsa.

3. Serve pork in tortillas topped with salsa.

Nutrition Facts (per serving = 2 tacos):

- Calories: 320

- Protein: 25g

- Carbohydrates: 35g

- Fat: 10g

- Fiber: 4g

- Sugar: 10g

22. Spiced Lamb and Couscous Salad

Servings: 4

Ingredients:

- 500g lamb steaks
- 1 cup couscous, cooked
- 1/2 cup cherry tomatoes, halved
- 1/4 cup feta cheese, crumbled
- 1/4 cup olives
- 2 tbsp olive oil
- Spices (cumin, coriander, paprika)
- Salt and pepper

Instructions:

1. Season lamb with spices, salt, and pepper. Grill until desired doneness.
2. Mix couscous, tomatoes, feta, olives, and olive oil.
3. Serve lamb on top of the couscous salad.

Nutrition Facts (per serving):

- Calories: 400
- Protein: 30g
- Carbohydrates: 25g
- Fat: 20g

- Fiber: 3g
- Sugar: 3g

23. Duck Breast with Orange Sauce

Servings: 4

Ingredients:

- 4 duck breasts
- 2 oranges, juiced
- 1 tbsp honey
- Salt and pepper

Instructions:

1. Score duck breast skin. Season with salt and pepper. Cook skin-side down until crispy.
2. Flip and cook the other side.
3. For the sauce, reduce orange juice and honey in a pan until thickened.
4. Serve duck breast with a drizzle of orange sauce.

Nutrition Facts (per serving = 1 duck breast with sauce):

- Calories: 380
- Protein: 25g
- Carbohydrates: 20g
- Fat: 20g
- Fiber: 2g
- Sugar: 18g

24. Beef and Mushroom Risotto

Servings: 4

Ingredients:

- 500g beef slices
- 1 cup Arborio rice
- 2 cups beef broth
- 1 cup mushrooms, sliced
- 1 onion, chopped
- 2 garlic cloves, minced
- 1 tbsp olive oil
- Parmesan cheese, grated
- Salt and pepper

Instructions:

1. In a pan, heat olive oil. Sauté onions and garlic.
2. Add beef and brown. Remove and set aside.
3. Add rice and stir for a minute. Gradually add broth while stirring until rice is cooked.
4. Add mushrooms and cooked beef. Season.
5. Serve with grated Parmesan on top.

Nutrition Facts (per serving):

- Calories: 420
- Protein: 30g

- Carbohydrates: 45g

- Fat: 15g

- Fiber: 2g

- Sugar: 3g

25. Chicken and Bean Chili

Servings: 4

Ingredients:

- 4 chicken breasts, cubed

- 1 can black beans, drained

- 1 can crushed tomatoes

- 1 onion, chopped

- 2 garlic cloves, minced

- 1 chili pepper, minced

- 2 tbsp olive oil

- Spices (cumin, coriander, paprika)

- Salt and pepper

Instructions:

1. In a pot, heat olive oil. Sauté onions, garlic, and chili pepper.

2. Add chicken and brown.

3. Add beans, crushed tomatoes, spices, salt, and pepper. Simmer until chicken is cooked.

Nutrition Facts (per serving):

- Calories: 340

- Protein: 35g

- Carbohydrates: 30g

- Fat: 10g

- Fiber: 8g

- Sugar: 6g

26. Pork and Cabbage Stir-fry

Servings: 4

Ingredients:

- 500g pork slices
- 4 cups cabbage, shredded
- 1 carrot, julienned
- 3 tbsp soy sauce
- 1 tbsp sesame oil
- 2 garlic cloves, minced

Instructions:

1. In a pan, heat sesame oil. Sauté garlic.
2. Add pork and cook until browned.
3. Add cabbage, carrot, and soy sauce. Stir-fry until vegetables are tender.

Nutrition Facts (per serving):

- Calories: 280
- Protein: 30g
- Carbohydrates: 10g
- Fat: 12g
- Fiber: 3g
- Sugar: 5g

27. Beef and Spinach Stuffed Eggplant

Servings: 4

Ingredients:

- 2 large eggplants, halved
- 500g lean ground beef
- 2 cups spinach, chopped
- 1 onion, chopped
- 2 garlic cloves, minced
- 1 tbsp olive oil
- Salt and pepper

Instructions:

1. Scoop out the flesh of the eggplants, leaving a shell.
2. In a pan, heat olive oil. Sauté onions and garlic.
3. Add beef and cook until browned. Add spinach and cook until wilted. Season.
4. Stuff the eggplant shells with the mixture. Bake at 375°F (190°C) for 25 minutes.

Nutrition Facts (per serving = 1 stuffed eggplant half):

- Calories: 350
- Protein: 30g
- Carbohydrates: 25g

- Fat: 15g

- Fiber: 10g

- Sugar: 10g

28. Salmon and Asparagus Foil Packs

Servings: 4

Ingredients:

- 4 salmon fillets
- 2 cups asparagus, trimmed
- 2 lemons, sliced
- 2 tbsp olive oil
- Salt, pepper, and dill

Instructions:

1. Place each salmon fillet on a foil piece. Top with asparagus and lemon slices.
2. Drizzle with olive oil and season. Wrap the foil.
3. Grill or bake at 375°F (190°C) for 20 minutes.

Nutrition Facts (per serving = 1 foil pack):

- Calories: 300
- Protein: 30g
- Carbohydrates: 5g
- Fat: 18g
- Fiber: 2g
- Sugar: 2g

29. Turkey and Cranberry Lettuce Wraps

Servings: 4

Ingredients:

- 500g ground turkey
- 1/2 cup dried cranberries
- 1/2 cup walnuts, chopped
- 1 apple, diced
- Romaine lettuce leaves
- 2 tbsp olive oil
- Salt and pepper

Instructions:

1. In a pan, heat olive oil. Cook turkey until browned.
2. Add cranberries, walnuts, and apple. Season.
3. Serve the mixture in lettuce leaves as wraps.

Nutrition Facts (per serving = 3 wraps):

- Calories: 340
- Protein: 25g
- Carbohydrates: 25g
- Fat: 18g
- Fiber: 4g
- Sugar: 18g

30. Lamb and Vegetable Curry

Servings: 4

Ingredients:

- 500g lamb cubes

- 2 cups mixed vegetables (carrots, peas, bell peppers)

- 1 can coconut milk

- 2 tbsp curry paste

- 1 onion, chopped

- 2 garlic cloves, minced

- 1 tbsp olive oil

Instructions:

1. In a pot, heat olive oil. Sauté onions and garlic.

2. Add lamb and brown.

3. Stir in curry paste. Add vegetables and coconut milk. Simmer until lamb is tender.

Nutrition Facts (per serving):

- Calories: 400

- Protein: 30g

- Carbohydrates: 20g

- Fat: 25g

- Fiber: 5g

- Sugar: 7g

31. Quinoa and Chicken Salad

Servings: 4

Ingredients:

- 2 cups cooked quinoa
- 2 grilled chicken breasts, diced
- 1 cup cherry tomatoes, halved
- 1 cucumber, diced
- 1/4 cup feta cheese
- Olive oil, lemon juice, salt, and pepper for dressing

Instructions:

1. Mix all ingredients in a large bowl.
2. Drizzle with dressing and toss.

Nutrition Facts (per serving):

- Calories: 310
- Protein: 28g
- Carbohydrates: 30g
- Fat: 8g
- Fiber: 5g
- Sugar: 4g

32. Sweet Potato and Lentil Curry

Servings: 4

Ingredients:

- 2 sweet potatoes, cubed
- 1 cup cooked lentils
- 1 onion, diced
- 2 garlic cloves, minced
- 1 can coconut milk
- 2 tbsp curry powder
- 1 tbsp olive oil
- Salt to taste

Instructions:

1. Sauté onion and garlic in olive oil until translucent.
2. Add sweet potatoes, lentils, coconut milk, and curry powder. Simmer until potatoes are tender.

Nutrition Facts (per serving):

- Calories: 320
- Protein: 12g
- Carbohydrates: 48g
- Fat: 10g
- Fiber: 10g

- Sugar: 8g

33. Steamed Fish with Ginger and Scallions

Servings: 4

Ingredients:

- 4 white fish fillets (like cod or halibut)
- 4 scallions, thinly sliced
- 2 inches ginger, julienned
- 2 tbsp soy sauce
- 1 tsp sesame oil

Instructions:

1. Steam fish fillets until cooked through.
2. Top with scallions and ginger. Drizzle with soy sauce and sesame oil.

Nutrition Facts (per serving):

- Calories: 180
- Protein: 30g
- Carbohydrates: 3g
- Fat: 4g
- Fiber: 1g
- Sugar: 1g

34. Roasted Veggie and Beef Stir-Fry

Servings: 4

Ingredients:

- 500g beef slices
- 4 cups mixed vegetables (bell peppers, broccoli, carrots)
- 3 tbsp low-sodium soy sauce
- 2 tbsp sesame oil
- 1 garlic clove, minced
- 1 tbsp ginger, minced

Instructions:

1. In a wok or large pan, heat sesame oil. Add garlic and ginger.
2. Add beef slices, cooking until browned.
3. Add veggies and stir until tender. Drizzle with soy sauce and serve.

Nutrition Facts (per serving):

- Calories: 320
- Protein: 28g
- Carbohydrates: 20g
- Fat: 12g
- Fiber: 5g
- Sugar: 6g

35. Spaghetti Squash and Turkey Meatballs

Servings: 4

Ingredients:

- 1 spaghetti squash, halved and seeds removed

- 500g ground turkey

- 1 can crushed tomatoes

- 1 onion, finely chopped

- 2 garlic cloves, minced

- 2 tbsp olive oil

- Salt, pepper, and Italian seasoning

Instructions:

1. Roast the spaghetti squash at 375°F (190°C) until tender. Scrape out the flesh with a fork.

2. Mix turkey with half of the onion, garlic, salt, and pepper. Form into meatballs.

3. In a pan, sauté the rest of the onion and garlic. Add crushed tomatoes and seasonings.

4. Add meatballs and simmer until cooked through. Serve over spaghetti squash.

Nutrition Facts (per serving):

- Calories: 360

- Protein: 28g

- Carbohydrates: 30g

- Fat: 12g

- Fiber: 8g

- Sugar: 10g

36. Herb-Crusted Pork Tenderloin

Servings: 4

Ingredients:

- 1 pork tenderloin
- 2 tbsp olive oil
- Mix of herbs (rosemary, thyme, parsley, minced)
- Salt and pepper

Instructions:

1. Rub the pork with olive oil, herbs, salt, and pepper.
2. Roast at 375°F (190°C) until cooked to desired doneness.

Nutrition Facts (per serving):

- Calories: 240
- Protein: 30g
- Carbohydrates: 0g
- Fat: 12g
- Fiber: 0g
- Sugar: 0g

37. Lamb Kebabs with Yogurt Sauce

Servings: 4

Ingredients:

- 500g lamb cubes

- 2 cups Greek yogurt

- 1 cucumber, finely chopped

- 2 garlic cloves, minced

- Lemon juice, olive oil, salt, pepper, and paprika

Instructions:

1. Skewer the lamb cubes. Drizzle with olive oil, lemon juice, salt, pepper, and paprika.

2. Grill until desired doneness.

3. Mix yogurt with cucumber and garlic. Serve as a sauce with the kebabs.

Nutrition Facts (per serving):

- Calories: 340

- Protein: 28g

- Carbohydrates: 8g

- Fat: 22g

- Fiber: 0g

- Sugar: 6g

38. Chicken and Vegetable Casserole

Servings: 4

Ingredients:

- 4 chicken breasts
- 4 cups mixed vegetables (zucchini, bell peppers, tomatoes)
- 1 can crushed tomatoes
- 1 onion, chopped
- 2 garlic cloves, minced
- 2 tbsp olive oil
- Salt, pepper, and herbs (basil, oregano)

Instructions:

1. Sauté onion and garlic in a casserole dish with olive oil.
2. Add chicken and brown on each side.
3. Add vegetables, crushed tomatoes, and seasonings. Cover and simmer until chicken is cooked through.

Nutrition Facts (per serving):

- Calories: 320
- Protein: 30g
- Carbohydrates: 20g
- Fat: 12g
- Fiber: 6g

- Sugar: 10g

39. Beef and Broccoli Teriyaki

Servings: 4

Ingredients:

- 500g beef slices
- 4 cups broccoli florets
- 1/4 cup teriyaki sauce
- 2 tbsp sesame oil
- 1 garlic clove, minced

Instructions:

1. In a wok, heat sesame oil. Add garlic and beef. Cook until browned.
2. Add broccoli and teriyaki sauce. Stir-fry until broccoli is tender.

Nutrition Facts (per serving):

- Calories: 300
- Protein: 28g
- Carbohydrates: 15g
- Fat: 14g
- Fiber: 4g
- Sugar: 6g

40. Salmon with Lemon-Dill Sauce

Servings: 4

Ingredients:

- 4 salmon fillets

- 2 tbsp olive oil

- Juice of 1 lemon

- 2 tbsp fresh dill, chopped

- Salt and pepper

Instructions:

1. Grill or pan-sear salmon with olive oil until cooked through.

2. Mix lemon juice, dill, salt, and pepper. Drizzle over salmon before serving.

Nutrition Facts (per serving):

- Calories: 310

- Protein: 28g

- Carbohydrates: 2g

- Fat: 20g

- Fiber: 0g

- Sugar: 1g

41. Garlic-Herb Roasted Chicken Thighs

Servings: 4

Ingredients:

- 8 chicken thighs
- 4 garlic cloves, minced
- Mix of herbs (rosemary, thyme, parsley, minced)
- 2 tbsp olive oil
- Salt and pepper

Instructions:

1. Rub chicken thighs with olive oil, garlic, herbs, salt, and pepper.
2. Roast at 375°F (190°C) until cooked through and skin is crispy.

Nutrition Facts (per serving):

- Calories: 360
- Protein: 30g
- Carbohydrates: 2g
- Fat: 26g
- Fiber: 0g
- Sugar: 0g

42. Grilled Tuna Steaks with Mango Salsa

Servings: 4

Ingredients:

- 4 tuna steaks
- 1 mango, diced
- 1 red bell pepper, diced
- 1/2 red onion, finely chopped
- Juice of 1 lime
- 1 tbsp fresh cilantro, chopped
- Salt and pepper

Instructions:

1. Grill tuna steaks to desired doneness.
2. Mix mango, bell pepper, onion, lime juice, cilantro, salt, and pepper. Serve as salsa over tuna.

Nutrition Facts (per serving):

- Calories: 240
- Protein: 30g
- Carbohydrates: 20g
- Fat: 4g
- Fiber: 3g
- Sugar: 15g

43. Turkey and Veggie Stuffed Peppers

Servings: 4

Ingredients:

- 4 bell peppers, tops removed and hollowed out
- 500g ground turkey
- 2 cups mixed veggies (zucchini, mushrooms, corn)
- 1 can crushed tomatoes
- 1 onion, chopped
- 2 garlic cloves, minced
- 2 tbsp olive oil
- Salt and pepper

Instructions:

1. Sauté onion and garlic in olive oil. Add turkey and cook until browned.
2. Add veggies and crushed tomatoes. Season.
3. Stuff bell peppers with the mixture. Roast at 375°F (190°C) until peppers are tender.

Nutrition Facts (per serving):

- Calories: 320
- Protein: 30g
- Carbohydrates: 30g

- Fat: 10g

- Fiber: 8g

- Sugar: 10g

44. Lamb Salad with Feta and Olives

Servings: 4

Ingredients:

- 500g grilled lamb slices
- 4 cups mixed salad greens
- 1 cup cherry tomatoes
- 1/2 cup feta cheese
- 1/2 cup kalamata olives
- Olive oil, lemon juice, salt, and pepper for dressing

Instructions:

1. Mix all ingredients in a large bowl.
2. Drizzle with dressing and toss.

Nutrition Facts (per serving):

- Calories: 400
- Protein: 30g
- Carbohydrates: 8g
- Fat: 28g
- Fiber: 3g
- Sugar: 4g

45. Rosemary Beef Skewers with Chimichurri

Servings: 4

Ingredients:

- 500g beef cubes

- 4 rosemary sprigs (as skewers)

- 1 cup fresh parsley, chopped

- 1/2 cup fresh cilantro, chopped

- 2 garlic cloves, minced

- 1/4 cup olive oil

- Juice of 1 lemon

- Salt and pepper

Instructions:

1. Skewer the beef cubes onto rosemary sprigs. Grill until desired doneness.

2. Mix parsley, cilantro, garlic, olive oil, lemon juice, salt, and pepper. Serve as chimichurri sauce with beef skewers.

Nutrition Facts (per serving):

- Calories: 350

- Protein: 28g

- Carbohydrates: 3g

- Fat: 26g

- Fiber: 1g

- Sugar: 1g

46. Chicken Caesar Salad with Yogurt Dressing

Servings: 4

Ingredients:

- 4 grilled chicken breasts, sliced

- 8 cups romaine lettuce, chopped

- 1/2 cup grated parmesan cheese

- For dressing: 1 cup Greek yogurt, 2 garlic cloves minced, juice of 1 lemon, 2 anchovy fillets (optional), salt, and pepper

Instructions:

1. Mix lettuce, chicken, and parmesan in a large bowl.

2. Blend dressing ingredients until smooth. Drizzle over salad.

Nutrition Facts (per serving):

- Calories: 320

- Protein: 40g

- Carbohydrates: 8g

- Fat: 12g

- Fiber: 3g

- Sugar: 4g

47. Pork and Pineapple Tacos

Servings: 4

Ingredients:

- 500g pork slices

- 1 cup pineapple chunks

- 8 small corn tortillas

- 1/2 red onion, finely chopped

- 1 jalapeño, sliced

- 1/4 cup fresh cilantro, chopped

- 2 limes, quartered

Instructions:

1. Grill pork until cooked. Set aside.

2. Grill pineapple chunks until slightly caramelized.

3. Assemble tacos using tortillas, pork, pineapple, onion, jalapeño, and cilantro. Serve with lime wedges.

Nutrition Facts (per serving - 2 tacos):

- Calories: 350

- Protein: 30g

- Carbohydrates: 35g

- Fat: 8g

- Fiber: 5g

- Sugar: 8g

48. Beef and Mushroom Lettuce Wraps

Servings: 4

Ingredients:

- 500g ground beef

- 2 cups mushrooms, finely chopped

- 8 large lettuce leaves (like Bibb or iceberg)

- 1 onion, finely chopped

- 2 garlic cloves, minced

- 2 tbsp low-sodium soy sauce

- 1 tsp sesame oil

Instructions:

1. Sauté onion and garlic in a pan with sesame oil. Add beef and cook until browned.

2. Add mushrooms and soy sauce. Cook until mushrooms are tender.

3. Spoon the mixture into lettuce leaves to serve as wraps.

Nutrition Facts (per serving - 2 wraps):

- Calories: 320

- Protein: 28g

- Carbohydrates: 8g

- Fat: 20g

- Fiber: 2g

- Sugar: 4g

49. Spicy Shrimp and Zucchini Noodles

Servings: 4

Ingredients:

- 500g shrimp, peeled and deveined

- 4 zucchinis, spiralized

- 2 tbsp olive oil

- 2 garlic cloves, minced

- 1 tsp chili flakes

- Salt and pepper

Instructions:

1. Sauté garlic and chili flakes in olive oil. Add shrimp and cook until pink.

2. Add zucchini noodles and stir until heated. Season with salt and pepper.

Nutrition Facts (per serving):

- Calories: 240

- Protein: 28g

- Carbohydrates: 10g

- Fat: 10g

- Fiber: 3g

- Sugar: 6g

50. Herbed Lamb and Roasted Veggie Bowls

Servings: 4

Ingredients:

- 500g lamb slices

- 4 cups mixed veggies (bell peppers, eggplant, cherry tomatoes)

- 2 tbsp olive oil

- Mix of herbs (rosemary, thyme, parsley, minced)

- Salt and pepper

Instructions:

1. Toss veggies in 1 tbsp olive oil, salt, pepper, and half of the herbs. Roast at 375°F (190°C) until tender.

2. Season lamb with remaining olive oil, herbs, salt, and pepper. Grill until desired doneness.

3. Serve lamb over roasted veggies in bowls.

Nutrition Facts (per serving):

- Calories: 360

- Protein: 28g

- Carbohydrates: 15g

- Fat: 22g

- Fiber: 5g

- Sugar: 7g

DAILY FOOD TRACKER

Date:

BREAKFAST	SNACKS	LUNCH	DINNER

TODAY'S WORKOUT

WATER INTAKE

NOTES

DAILY FOOD TRACKER

Date:

BREAKFAST	SNACKS	LUNCH	DINNER

TODAY'S WORKOUT

WATER INTAKE

NOTES

DAILY FOOD TRACKER

Date:

BREAKFAST	SNACKS	LUNCH	DINNER

TODAY'S WORKOUT

WATER INTAKE

NOTES

DAILY FOOD TRACKER

Date:

BREAKFAST	SNACKS	LUNCH	DINNER

TODAY'S WORKOUT

WATER INTAKE

NOTES

DAILY FOOD TRACKER

Date:

BREAKFAST	SNACKS	LUNCH	DINNER

TODAY'S WORKOUT

WATER INTAKE

NOTES

DAILY FOOD TRACKER

Date:

BREAKFAST	SNACKS	LUNCH	DINNER

TODAY'S WORKOUT

WATER INTAKE

NOTES

DAILY FOOD TRACKER

Date:

BREAKFAST	SNACKS	LUNCH	DINNER

TODAY'S WORKOUT

WATER INTAKE

NOTES

DAILY FOOD TRACKER

Date:

BREAKFAST	SNACKS	LUNCH	DINNER

TODAY'S WORKOUT

WATER INTAKE

NOTES

DAILY FOOD TRACKER

Date:

BREAKFAST	SNACKS	LUNCH	DINNER

TODAY'S WORKOUT

WATER INTAKE

NOTES

DAILY FOOD TRACKER

Date:

BREAKFAST	SNACKS	LUNCH	DINNER

TODAY'S WORKOUT

WATER INTAKE

NOTES

DAILY FOOD TRACKER

Date:

BREAKFAST	SNACKS	LUNCH	DINNER

TODAY'S WORKOUT

WATER INTAKE

NOTES

DAILY FOOD TRACKER

Date:

BREAKFAST	SNACKS	LUNCH	DINNER

TODAY'S WORKOUT

WATER INTAKE

NOTES

DAILY FOOD TRACKER

Date:

BREAKFAST	SNACKS	LUNCH	DINNER

TODAY'S WORKOUT

WATER INTAKE

NOTES

DAILY FOOD TRACKER

Date:

BREAKFAST	SNACKS	LUNCH	DINNER

TODAY'S WORKOUT

WATER INTAKE

NOTES

DAILY FOOD TRACKER

Date:

BREAKFAST	SNACKS	LUNCH	DINNER

TODAY'S WORKOUT

WATER INTAKE

NOTES

DAILY FOOD TRACKER

Date:

BREAKFAST	SNACKS	LUNCH	DINNER

TODAY'S WORKOUT

WATER INTAKE

NOTES

DAILY FOOD TRACKER

Date:

BREAKFAST	SNACKS	LUNCH	DINNER

TODAY'S WORKOUT

WATER INTAKE

NOTES

DAILY FOOD TRACKER

Date:

BREAKFAST	SNACKS	LUNCH	DINNER

TODAY'S WORKOUT

WATER INTAKE

NOTES

DAILY FOOD TRACKER

Date:

BREAKFAST	SNACKS	LUNCH	DINNER

TODAY'S WORKOUT

WATER INTAKE

NOTES

DAILY FOOD TRACKER

Date:

BREAKFAST	SNACKS	LUNCH	DINNER

TODAY'S WORKOUT

WATER INTAKE

NOTES

DAILY FOOD TRACKER

Date:

BREAKFAST	SNACKS	LUNCH	DINNER

TODAY'S WORKOUT

WATER INTAKE

NOTES

DAILY FOOD TRACKER

Date:

BREAKFAST	SNACKS	LUNCH	DINNER

TODAY'S WORKOUT

WATER INTAKE

NOTES

DAILY FOOD TRACKER

Date:

BREAKFAST	SNACKS	LUNCH	DINNER

TODAY'S WORKOUT

WATER INTAKE

NOTES

DAILY FOOD TRACKER

Date:

BREAKFAST	SNACKS	LUNCH	DINNER

TODAY'S WORKOUT

WATER INTAKE

NOTES

DAILY FOOD TRACKER

Date:

BREAKFAST	SNACKS	LUNCH	DINNER

TODAY'S WORKOUT

WATER INTAKE

NOTES

DAILY FOOD TRACKER

Date:

BREAKFAST	SNACKS	LUNCH	DINNER

TODAY'S WORKOUT

WATER INTAKE

NOTES

DAILY FOOD TRACKER

Date:

BREAKFAST	SNACKS	LUNCH	DINNER

TODAY'S WORKOUT

WATER INTAKE

NOTES

DAILY FOOD TRACKER

Date:

BREAKFAST	SNACKS	LUNCH	DINNER

TODAY'S WORKOUT

WATER INTAKE

NOTES

DAILY FOOD TRACKER

Date:

BREAKFAST	SNACKS	LUNCH	DINNER

TODAY'S WORKOUT

WATER INTAKE

NOTES

DAILY FOOD TRACKER

Date:

BREAKFAST	SNACKS	LUNCH	DINNER

TODAY'S WORKOUT

WATER INTAKE

NOTES

DAILY FOOD TRACKER

Date:

BREAKFAST	SNACKS	LUNCH	DINNER

TODAY'S WORKOUT

WATER INTAKE

NOTES

DAILY FOOD TRACKER

Date:

BREAKFAST	SNACKS	LUNCH	DINNER

TODAY'S WORKOUT

WATER INTAKE

NOTES

DAILY FOOD TRACKER

Date:

BREAKFAST	SNACKS	LUNCH	DINNER

TODAY'S WORKOUT

WATER INTAKE

NOTES

DAILY FOOD TRACKER

Date:

BREAKFAST	SNACKS	LUNCH	DINNER

TODAY'S WORKOUT	WATER INTAKE

NOTES

DAILY FOOD TRACKER

Date:

BREAKFAST	SNACKS	LUNCH	DINNER

TODAY'S WORKOUT

WATER INTAKE

NOTES

DAILY FOOD TRACKER

Date:

BREAKFAST	SNACKS	LUNCH	DINNER

TODAY'S WORKOUT

WATER INTAKE

NOTES

DAILY FOOD TRACKER

Date:

BREAKFAST	SNACKS	LUNCH	DINNER

TODAY'S WORKOUT

WATER INTAKE

NOTES

DAILY FOOD TRACKER

Date:

BREAKFAST	SNACKS	LUNCH	DINNER

TODAY'S WORKOUT

WATER INTAKE

NOTES

DAILY FOOD TRACKER

Date:

BREAKFAST	SNACKS	LUNCH	DINNER

TODAY'S WORKOUT

WATER INTAKE

NOTES

DAILY FOOD TRACKER

Date:

BREAKFAST	SNACKS	LUNCH	DINNER

TODAY'S WORKOUT

WATER INTAKE

NOTES

DAILY FOOD TRACKER

Date:

BREAKFAST	SNACKS	LUNCH	DINNER

TODAY'S WORKOUT

WATER INTAKE

NOTES

DAILY FOOD TRACKER

Date:

BREAKFAST	SNACKS	LUNCH	DINNER

TODAY'S WORKOUT

WATER INTAKE

NOTES

DAILY FOOD TRACKER

Date:

BREAKFAST	SNACKS	LUNCH	DINNER

TODAY'S WORKOUT

WATER INTAKE

NOTES

DAILY FOOD TRACKER

Date:

BREAKFAST	SNACKS	LUNCH	DINNER

TODAY'S WORKOUT

WATER INTAKE

NOTES

DAILY FOOD TRACKER

Date:

BREAKFAST	SNACKS	LUNCH	DINNER

TODAY'S WORKOUT

WATER INTAKE

NOTES

DAILY FOOD TRACKER

Date:

BREAKFAST	SNACKS	LUNCH	DINNER

TODAY'S WORKOUT

WATER INTAKE

NOTES

DAILY FOOD TRACKER

Date:

BREAKFAST	SNACKS	LUNCH	DINNER

TODAY'S WORKOUT

WATER INTAKE

NOTES

DAILY FOOD TRACKER

Date:

BREAKFAST	SNACKS	LUNCH	DINNER

TODAY'S WORKOUT

WATER INTAKE

NOTES

DAILY FOOD TRACKER

Date:

BREAKFAST	SNACKS	LUNCH	DINNER

TODAY'S WORKOUT

WATER INTAKE

NOTES

DAILY FOOD TRACKER

Date:

BREAKFAST	SNACKS	LUNCH	DINNER

TODAY'S WORKOUT

WATER INTAKE

NOTES

DAILY FOOD TRACKER

Date:

BREAKFAST	SNACKS	LUNCH	DINNER

TODAY'S WORKOUT

WATER INTAKE

NOTES

DAILY FOOD TRACKER

Date:

BREAKFAST	SNACKS	LUNCH	DINNER

TODAY'S WORKOUT

WATER INTAKE

NOTES

DAILY FOOD TRACKER

Date:

BREAKFAST	SNACKS	LUNCH	DINNER

TODAY'S WORKOUT

WATER INTAKE

NOTES

DAILY FOOD TRACKER

Date:

BREAKFAST	SNACKS	LUNCH	DINNER

TODAY'S WORKOUT

WATER INTAKE

NOTES

DAILY FOOD TRACKER

Date:

BREAKFAST	SNACKS	LUNCH	DINNER

TODAY'S WORKOUT

WATER INTAKE

NOTES

DAILY FOOD TRACKER

Date:

BREAKFAST	SNACKS	LUNCH	DINNER

TODAY'S WORKOUT

WATER INTAKE

NOTES

DAILY FOOD TRACKER

Date:

BREAKFAST	SNACKS	LUNCH	DINNER

TODAY'S WORKOUT

WATER INTAKE

NOTES

DAILY FOOD TRACKER

Date:

BREAKFAST	SNACKS	LUNCH	DINNER

TODAY'S WORKOUT

WATER INTAKE

NOTES

DAILY FOOD TRACKER

Date:

BREAKFAST	SNACKS	LUNCH	DINNER

TODAY'S WORKOUT

WATER INTAKE

NOTES

DAILY FOOD TRACKER

Date:

BREAKFAST	SNACKS	LUNCH	DINNER

TODAY'S WORKOUT

WATER INTAKE

NOTES

DAILY FOOD TRACKER

Date:

BREAKFAST	SNACKS	LUNCH	DINNER

TODAY'S WORKOUT

WATER INTAKE

NOTES

DAILY FOOD TRACKER

Date:

BREAKFAST	SNACKS	LUNCH	DINNER

TODAY'S WORKOUT

WATER INTAKE

NOTES

DAILY FOOD TRACKER

Date:

BREAKFAST	SNACKS	LUNCH	DINNER

TODAY'S WORKOUT

WATER INTAKE

NOTES

DAILY FOOD TRACKER

Date:

BREAKFAST	SNACKS	LUNCH	DINNER

TODAY'S WORKOUT

WATER INTAKE

NOTES

DAILY FOOD TRACKER

Date:

BREAKFAST	SNACKS	LUNCH	DINNER

TODAY'S WORKOUT

WATER INTAKE

NOTES

DAILY FOOD TRACKER

Date:

BREAKFAST	SNACKS	LUNCH	DINNER

TODAY'S WORKOUT

WATER INTAKE

NOTES

DAILY FOOD TRACKER

Date:

BREAKFAST	SNACKS	LUNCH	DINNER

TODAY'S WORKOUT

WATER INTAKE

NOTES